Sobhi Mleyhi
Tarek sendi
Raouf Denguir

Surgery for congenital heart disease in adulthood

Sobhi Mleyhi
Tarek sendi
Raouf Denguir

Surgery for congenital heart disease in adulthood

Surgery for congenital heart disease

ScienciaScripts

Cover image: www.ingimage.com

This book is a translation from the original published under ISBN 978-620-3-42384-6.

Publisher:
Sciencia Scripts
is a trademark of
Dodo Books Indian Ocean Ltd., member of the OmniScriptum S.R.L Publishing group
str. A.Russo 15, of. 61, Chisinau-2068, Republic of Moldova Europe
Printed at: see last page
ISBN: 978-620-4-03356-3

List of abbreviations

CCC: cyanogenic congenital heart disease

NCCD: non-cyanogenic congenital heart disease

TGV: transposition of large vessels

T4F: Tetralogy of Fallot

PI : pulmonary insufficiency

PR: pulmonary shrinkage

PVR: pulmonary valve replacement

VD: right ventricle

LV: left ventricle

PR: pulmonary narrowing

TAC: common arterial trunk

VDDI: double outlet right ventricle

CoA: coarctation of the aorta

ECG: electrocardiogram

HR: rhythmic holter

TTE: trans thoracic ultrasound

MRI: magnetic resonance imaging

CT: computed tomography

CEC: extracorporeal circulation

APT: pulmonary artery trunk

Gd: gradient

AHA: American Heart Association

RVSP: right ventricular systolic pressure

ESC : European society of Cardiology

PSA: pulmonary atresia with intact septum

APSO : open septum pulmonary atresia

VIC: ventricular septal defect

AIC: atrial septal defect

AVC: atrioventricular canal

PCPD: percutaneous pulmonary dilatation

REV: repair at the ventricular stage

NYHA: New York Heart Association

ACFA: complete arrhythmia by atrial fibrillation

ESA: atrial extra systole

VT: ventricular tachycardia

ESV: extra ventricular systole

AVB: atrioventricular block

BBD: right branch block

RDVD: right ventricular end-diastolic diameter

LVEDD: left ventricular end-diastolic diameter

TAPSE: tricuspid annular plane systolic excursion

LVEF: left ventricular ejection fraction

IT: tricuspid insufficiency

MI: mitral insufficiency

IAo: aortic insufficiency

RVEDV: right ventricular end-diastolic volume

RVTSV: right ventricular end-systolic volume

RVEF: right ventricular ejection fraction

CEC: extracorporeal circulation

CEE: external electric shock

VF: ventricular fibrillation

MAPCA: major aorto-pulmonary collateral arteries

I. Introduction:

Congenital heart disease (CHD) is defined as any malformation of the heart present at birth. They are due either to a developmental defect or to the abnormal persistence of structures normally present during fetal life. They are the most frequent congenital malformations and affect nearly 1% of births [1].

Several segmental classifications have been proposed, based on the division of the heart into three main segments: atria (right and left), ventricles (right and left), and large vessels (aorta and pulmonary artery). The pathophysiological classification remains the most commonly used in most cases. Indeed, heart diseases with the same clinical appearance often result in the same hemodynamic consequences. Two main groups have been considered:

- Cyanogenic congenital heart disease.
- Non-cyanogenic congenital heart disease.

Since the advent of congenital heart surgery, the epidemiology of patients with CC has been transformed. Indeed, surgeries have been developed for CC previously considered irreparable. At the same time, advances in prenatal diagnosis have had little impact on the number of live births of children with heart defects. As a result, the population of adults with congenital heart disease, whether operated or not, is growing and it is considered that currently about 85% of patients reach adolescence and adulthood [2]. Thus, in developed countries CC is becoming the leading cause of heart disease in young adults [3-4].

Not long ago, congenital heart disease was primarily a pediatric condition. Because of the decrease in pediatric mortality of multifactorial origin, adult patients with congenital heart disease represent a new patient population that is constantly increasing in number and complexity and requires specialized management. Surgery for these heart diseases in adulthood has particular characteristics that differentiate it from congenital heart surgery in children and from surgery for acquired heart disease. In developed countries, the specific management of this population in referral centers has contributed to the improvement of surgical results in terms of mortality and subsequent quality of life.

II. Epidemiological characteristics:

Since the advent of cardiac surgery, and in particular congenital heart surgery, the epidemiology of patients with congenital heart disease has been transformed. Indeed, this pathology has become the leading cause of heart disease in young adults and expectant mothers in Western countries. There are several reasons for the increase in the number and complexity of cases of adult patients with CC undergoing cardiac surgery[5, 6] :

- ✓ First, more and more CC patients are now surviving into adulthood, including patients with complex disease [7].
- ✓ Second, the increase in age of this cohort implies an increase in the percentage of patients requiring surgery or reoperation among them [8, 9].
- ✓ Third, there has been a recent trend to operate on mildly symptomatic or asymptomatic patients to improve their prognosis. For example, pulmonary valve replacement after repair of tetralogy of Fallot is currently advocated in patients with severe pulmonary insufficiency and right ventricular dilatation independent of symptoms i.e. before clinical decompensation [10].

Similar to data previously reported in other studies [11-15], repair of septal defects, right heart, and left heart defects remain the most common in this population; with the finding of an increase in the number of patients requiring repair of right and left heart lesions contrasting with a decrease in surgical repair of septal defects. One possible explanation for such a trend stems from recent advances in interventional cardiology with the decrease in specific surgical procedures such as septal defect closure, PCAs and coarctation cure [16-19]. Another factor contributing to the decrease in septal defect closure is the increasing number of patients diagnosed and treated early in childhood due to advances in exploratory techniques.

1. Age:

The mean age at surgery that has been reported in the literature ranges from 24 ± 10.3 years for the series of Talwar S et al [12] (which included all patients ≥ 13 years) to 40 years [28 - 51 years] in the series of Karsenty et al [20]. The highest mean age (57.5 years) was reported in a series by Agarwal et al in the United States including all patients hospitalized for GUCH whether for surgery or not [21]. To the best of our knowledge, the oldest patient operated on for congenital heart disease was 87 years old at the time of closure of an aged ASD [22].
However, the mean age of complex CC was lower than the average (29 years) [23]. Nevertheless, a higher mean age of complex CC has been noted in other studies, notably that of Giannakoulas et al. in Greece with a mean age of 35 years [24] and in the CONCOR Registry (the CONgenital CORvitia (CONCOR) databa) in the Netherlands of 53 years [25].
The most represented age group was under 25 years in the series of Engelfriet et al [22] involving 79% of the patients.

2. Gender:

CCs operated on in adulthood, all types combined, were more frequent in women. For example, the sex ratio F/H was 1.4 in the series of Aleman-Ortiz et al [26], but almost equal to 1 in the series of Giannakoulas et al (F/H=1.08) [21]. For Engelfriet and colleagues [22], the proportion of women differed by type of defect, In aged AICs, 67% of patients were women compared to only 39% in CoA and large vessel transpositions (LVT). In addition, some studies have shown that the sex ratio tends to be reversed (F/H<1) by increasing the rate of men in the CC population, such as in the study by Diller et al (F/H=0.93) [27] and the study by Van Bulck et al [28].

III. History of the disease:

The surgical approach to congenital heart disease in adulthood in developing countries is different from that in developed countries. The diagnosis was made late in life. The high number of adolescents and adults with various native heart diseases reflects the lack of access to screening and sometimes surgery during childhood. By the time they arrive at adult cardiovascular surgery services, they are already at the stage of complications described in studies done in similar states [29-31], and this also suggests that a significant number of patients may miss the opportunity for optimal surgical intervention. M N Awori and colleagues [31] concluded that parental income appears to influence the medical management of patients but not parental education. Thus, patients with CC discovered in adulthood usually had simple, undetectable congenital heart defects or complex cyanotic defects that can still be compensated for allowing them to achieve a good quality of life until the onset of age-related complications [32, 33].

1. History of previous cardiac surgery:

The population of adult congenital heart patients is growing rapidly with a current estimated prevalence of 3,000 per million inhabitants, i.e. more than 150,000 people in France [34]. Most of them have been operated in childhood, but some have a native heart disease that allows them to live until adulthood. However, these patients cannot be considered cured. They frequently have residual lesions or sequelae at a distance from the surgical correction with a hemodynamic and very often rhythmic impact. Some authors [34-36] have proposed a classification of adults with CC based on the history of their disease (operated or not in childhood).

a) **Palliative surgery:**

Palliative techniques still have an important place, when definitive repair is not feasible at a given time or when complete cure has a significantly higher mortality risk [37, 38]. Their aim is to regulate pulmonary flow:

or excessive: by banding of the pulmonary artery trunk

- or insufficient: by a systemic-pulmonary shunt of the Blalock or De Leval type, or cavo-uni or bipulmonary anastomosis (Glenn) or the Fontan procedure [39].

➢ **Systemic-pulmonary shunt:**

The principle of the Blalock Taussig procedure is to increase pulmonary flow by creating a shunt between a subclavian artery and the homolateral branch of the pulmonary artery [40]. Initially the shunt was created by anastomosing the subclavian artery directly with a branch of the pulmonary artery. The procedure was modified by S. FRANK REDO and ROGER R. ECKER [41] by interposing a prosthetic tube between the two arteries. The main advantage of the modified Blalock is the possibility of calibration according to the age of the patient. It also allows preservation of the arterial supply to the upper limb. However, the anastomosis remains of great interest in irregular forms of tetralogies of Fallot with hypoplasia of the pulmonary tree. The procedure not only allows the pulmonary artery and its branches to be enlarged but also allows the pulmonary annulus to grow [42].

➢ **Pulmonary artery cerclage:**

The first description of pulmonary artery banding was made by Muller and Dammann at the University of California in 1952 [43]. Over the years, several techniques have been developed to adjust the cerclage circumference [44] :

-adjustable strapping was applied in 1972,

Percutaneous adjustment of the strapping band in 1986

and the FLOWATCH® (figure 1) (telemetry control) in recent years.

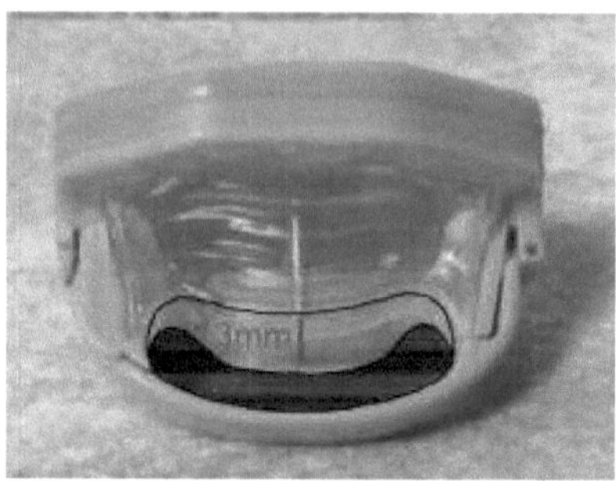

Figure 1: FLOWATCH

- **Partial cavo-pulmonary bypass (Glenn procedure):**

In 1958, William Glenn created the anastomosis between the right pulmonary artery and the superior vena cava without extracorporeal circulation [45]. There are several technical modalities for performing the bi-directional shunt: with or without extracorporeal circulation [46].

b) Reconstructive surgery:

- **The complete cure :**

Cono-truncal pathology is the embryological entity that groups together the different congenital heart diseases following a malformation of the conal septum. However, despite the common origin of these cardiopathies, they remain distinct pathophysiological entities in terms of their clinical manifestations, prognosis and the type of repair they require. The degree of complexity of their complete cures is very variable. It can range from simple commissurotomy during pulmonary narrowing to trans-annular patching or tube interposition. The subsequent use of a pulmonary valve replacement (PVR) depends much more on the procedure performed on the LV outflow tract and more precisely on the pulmonary annulus than on the type of conotruncal heart disease itself. When the complete cure includes an enlargement of the pulmonary annulus, the rate of revision for PVR after 25 years varies between

7.3 % [47] and 10 % [48]. This figure increases with the duration of follow-up, reaching 36% after 40 years [49]. When the integrity of the annulus is preserved, the rate of revision is lower, around 5% at 20 years [50].

The high rate of annular enlargement at complete cure is explained by the high percentage of patients with T4F. This malformation constitutes 8% of congenital heart disease, and annular pulmonary stenosis is almost always present, which makes the use of annular enlargement just as frequent. This high rate of annular enlargement can also be explained by the therapeutic strategy of some teams which consists in restoring the annulus to a surface area adapted to the body surface of the patient, whereas other teams tolerate stenoses judged to be moderate, considering the benefit provided by the annular cleft to be negligible compared to its disadvantages [50].

2. The complete post-cure follow-up:

The recommendations for congenital heart disease indicate that follow-up should be carried out in reference centers by physicians accustomed to the management of these pathologies, without specifying the frequency or the examinations to be performed [51]. This is due to the particularity of each patient and the need to personalize the follow-up.

IV. Surgery for congenital heart disease in adulthood:

1. Incidence and type of surgery:

Most surgeries are reparative (86%) and 58% of patients undergo surgery for the first time in adulthood. These patients are mostly adults with an atrial septal defect [52, 53].

Furthermore, Interestingly, with a growing population, reoperations are expected to outnumber primary repairs in adulthood [54]. However, as noted above, we believe that the increasing number of interventional procedures performed by cardiologists (ie, pulmonary valve implantation, coarctation repair, and percutaneous closure of CIAs and PCAs) appears to keep their numbers fairly stable over time [55,56].

According to the German registry, over a 15-year follow-up, 20% of patients with congenital heart disease require surgery in adulthood and almost 40% are re-interventions [8].

The most frequent re-interventions are those performed on the right ejection pathway, such as pulmonary valvulation in tetralogy of Fallot [48, 57, 58] and the replacement of a degenerated or insufficiently sized LV-AP tube. However, the increase in the number of re-interventions and the increase in the age of the patients at the time of the procedure make the surgical procedures sometimes complex [59].

2. Time between complete cure and re-intervention:

- For patients operated on for VAD, the average time between complete cure and reoperation for severe mitral insufficiency is 9.3 years. The indication for reoperation is mainly severe mitral insufficiency or left ventricular outflow tract obstruction [60-62]. The risk factors for reoperation for mitral insufficiency are congestive heart failure preoperatively and the finding of moderate or significant mitral insufficiency postoperatively [63].

In the majority of cases a second mitral plasty is feasible [64-78]. However, Stulak et al [62] described a rate of only 52% mitral plasty in their cohort of 92 patients.

- For conotruncal pathologies, the average time between complete cure and pulmonary valvulation varies from 19 to 29.4 years [69-71]. A study by Kogon B. et al [72] of 107 patients was interested in identifying factors that could affect the time from complete cure to PVR. Two factors were isolated: male sex and the diameter of the pulmonary artery branches. Both parameters would decrease this time. Neither the fraction of regurgitation nor the age of the complete cure had any influence on this delay.

3. Clinical data:

The clinical presentations of congenital heart disease vary depending on the type of defect, severity, and age at diagnosis. In adults, symptoms may include dyspnea, murmur, chest pain, palpitations, syncope, or even signs of heart failure [73].

Dyspnea is the most frequent functional complaint and most often the first complaint. It is also the main reason for patients to consult. Although its collection and staging are biased by its examiner-dependent nature, it is still of major interest and is sometimes the only symptom reported in the literature [74-76].

Chest pain is a very subjective sign that cannot be quantified and is difficult to attribute to the course of heart disease in these patients. Palpitations and right ventricular dysfunction were better explored, objectified, and quantified by rhythmic holter and cardiac imaging than by simple questioning or physical examination.

Syncope is a very important symptom but only when it is attributed to a severe rhythm disorder [77,78].

4. Paraclinical examinations:

Surveillance, operative indication and postoperative follow-up are based almost exclusively on the data of the clinical examination and the TTE. Exploration by CT scan, angiography or scintigraphy is most often performed only when non-invasive examinations cannot provide the necessary data. No single imaging modality could provide all the anatomical and hemodynamic information, and the exploration had to be personalized according to the patient's clinical condition and the rapidity of progression of his heart disease [79].

a) Electrical evaluation:

Its simplicity and availability are its major assets. This examination makes it possible to identify serious paroxysmal electrical abnormalities (VT, VF), to explain certain patient complaints, and may constitute in itself an indication for surgery.

The occurrence of arrhythmias is a well-known complication during the course of congenital heart disease in adulthood often leading to hospitalization. Indeed, the risk of arrhythmias is increased due to dilatation of the right atrium, myocardial hypertrophy, and previous surgical interventions [80]. Atrial fibrillation is the most frequent rhythmic complication [81].

In the aged CIA group, Mark Kotowycz and colleagues reported a 19% incidence of ACFA in 718 patients aged 18 to 75 years [82].

Numerous studies [83-86] have shown that QRS duration (≥180 ms) or change in QRS duration identifies patients at higher risk for ventricular rhythm disturbance, syncope, exercise intolerance, and ventricular dysfunction or sudden death. This makes ECGs not only a diagnostic tool but also a means of screening and risk stratification.

Sudden death from ventricular rhythm disturbance is the second most common cause of death in these patients after ventricular dysfunction [84]. Currently, patients at risk of SVR are screened by electrophysiological examinationsdetermine the threshold at which these patients are likely to have such disorders and to subsequently indicate defibrillator implantation [85].

b) TTE and MRI:

i. Right Heart Assessment:

The anatomic and hemodynamic evaluation of patients with CC is a real challenge. Two main examinations allow the study of the DV: TTE and MRI. Each of them has its advantages and indications.

Evaluation of pulmonary valve disease:

- ✓ Pulmonary insufficiency**:** MRI is the reference for the evaluation of pulmonary insufficiency. The latter is considered significant when the regurgitation fraction is ≥ 25% and it is considered severe when this fraction is ≥ 40%. However, the use of TTE for the evaluation of this parameter is more difficult. Some use the "pressure half time" with a severity threshold of 100 ms or the ratio between the diameter of the regurgitated jet and that of the pulmonary annulus with a severity threshold varying between 50 and 70%. Some studies have compared the regurgitation fraction assessed by MRI to the ratio of regurgitation duration to total diastolic time assessed by TTE. A threshold value of 0.77 provided high sensitivity and specificity for identifying patients with significant PI.
- ✓ Pulmonary stenosis**:** The evaluation of pulmonary stenosis must be both hemodynamic and anatomic. The particularity of MRI is that it is more accurate in the case of staged stenoses frequently found in patients whose complete cure required the placement of a valved tube.

✦ Role of TTE in the evaluation of the VD and pulmonary tree:

The TST is considered the gold standard examination. Its low cost and availability made it a constant step in every consultation.

- ✓ Anatomical evaluation: The search for infundibular aneurysms, the measurement of the thickness of the wall of the VD, the localization of possible residual pulmonary valve tissue as well as the complete evaluation of the pulmonary tree have a direct impact on the surgical technique to be used. In patients under ten years of age, sub-costal windows are of good resolution and offer an anatomical evaluation quite similar to that provided by angiography. But beyond this age, the quality and accuracy of the data provided by TTE decreases.
- ✓ Hemodynamic assessment: European and American scientific societies recommend that no single parameter should be used to assess LV systolic function (e.g., LV surface shortening fraction (SF) and tricuspid annulus lateral shift (TAPSE)). These different variables are proven for ischemic heart disease but are not proven for the assessment of right ventricular function [87]. TAPSE was the most commonly used variable to assess right systolic function. The threshold of 15 mm offered a sensitivity of 100% and a specificity of 41% for LV dysfunction [88].

✦ Role of MRI in the evaluation of the DV and pulmonary tree:

Cardiac MRI is currently the reference examination for the follow-up of patients who have had a complete cure [89- 93]. There is not yet a consensus on the frequency of this monitoring but it should be personalized according to the initial procedure performed, the patient's clinical status and the preoperative imaging data [94].

✓ Anatomical and hemodynamic assessment of the DV: The assessment of the anatomy of the DV and its systolic function are very dependent on each other. The two most important parameters to measure are the volume of the DV and its ejection fraction.

✓ *DV volume*: Numerous studies have attempted to determine the parameters to be monitored and the appropriate dilatation threshold to be instituted to indicate surgery (Table 1). For the majority of them, VTDVDi is the primary endpoint [100] but VTSVDi is also used.

Table 1: VTDVDi threshold indicating PVR according to the literature

Study	**Oosterhof [94]**	**Frigiola [95]**	**Buechel [96]**	**Geva [97]**	**Therrien [98]**	**Lee [99]**
[Year - Sample Size]	2007-71	2008-71	2005-20	2013-85	2005-17	2012-170
Threshold of VTDVDi (ml/m²sc)	160	150	150	150	170	163

It is important to note that none of these authors found a threshold beyond which the size of the DV no longer decreases but the improvement is most significant with these values.

✓ *DV ejection fraction:* Measurement of the DV ejection fraction requires consideration of:

*The size of the patches used for IVC closure and pulmonary annulus enlargement.

The anatomical limits of the papillary muscles and those of the most important trabeculations.

*Limitations of the endocardium of the VD.

*The volumes regurgitated by the pulmonary and tricuspid valve.
It should also be noted that these data are operator dependent. The contouring of the heart chambers is done manually.

- ✓ Anatomical assessment of the pulmonary tree:

Anatomical evaluation of the pulmonary tree by MRI allows mainly the study of its complex relationships with adjacent structures. This modality also offers an accurate measurement of the degree and extent of stenoses, particularly when they are staged. Its results are similar to those provided by angiography without being as invasive.

Correlation between TTE and MRI:

According to Koestenberger [100] the global right ventricular function evaluated by TAPSE did not correlate with the FEVD measured by MRI. However, according to another study by Promphan et al [91], TAPSE offers results that are comparable to those of MRI with a significance of $P < 0.01$.
According to the American Society of Echocardiography, follow-up of patients by TTE alone during the first decade after repair would be sufficient. This is justified by the stability of patients during this period and the mandatory use of general anesthesia before the age of 10 years. After this age, regular use of MRI becomes possible, especially as the increase in patient body mass reduces the acoustic windows, which minimizes the quality of the ultrasound results.

Tricuspid valve disease:

Tricuspid insufficiency is frequently present after complete cure of T4F. Its mechanisms include:

- ✓ Deterioration of the anteroseptal commissure structure due to the patching of the IVC closure and due to detachment of the septal leaflet of the valve.

- ✓ Enlargement of the annulus and change in the geometry of the subvalvular apparatus as a result of dilatation of the DV.
- ✓ Injuries caused by an implanted defibrillator or by endocarditis.
- ✓ Rarely, IT can be of congenital origin.

Many parameters can be used to evaluate the severity of the TI such as the Doppler signal intensity or the diameter of the regurgitated jet. Zoghbi et al [101] considered vena contracta to be the most reliable parameter and defined a value of 0.7 cm higher to speak of severe TIA.

ii. *Left heart assessment:*

LV systolic function is a very important prognostic factor. Its alteration is associated with an increased risk of early mortality. The evaluation of this function by the usual techniques assumes a geometrical shape and homogeneous contraction of the LV, but in our case this is not always the case. The important dilatation of the VD tends to decrease the symmetrical character of the LV. Subsequently, the measurement of LV dimensions by 3D TTE is preferred to that by 2D. In a study of 413 cases, Diller et al showed that nongeometric indices of LV longitudinal function assessments, particularly mitral annulus plane motion (analogous to TAPSE), are significantly associated with higher rates of major complications.

It allows a complete assessment of the left atrioventricular valve (AVV) as well as the aortic valve. It also allows follow-up before and after repair of an AVC or Ebstein's anomaly, by evaluating the mechanisms of valve leaks. Complex heart diseases such as double outlet right ventricle are particularly suitable for 3D analysis to predict surgical strategy.

iii. *Septal assessment and associated anomalies:*

Echocardiography is a cardinal imaging modality to determine the position of the septal defect as well as its size and relationship to adjacent structures. It also provides prognostic information by measuring shunts. In the long term, large septal defects can lead to pulmonary hypertension reversing the left-to-right shunt [102].

TEE allows the timing and type of intervention (surgery or percutaneous intervention) to be determined [103] and postoperatively allows the location of the closure device and residual shunts to be assessed [102]. Knowing that, TEE remains more efficient in the exploration of these residual defects [104].

Two-dimensional echocardiography allows the study of valvular anomalies associated with supra-sternal coarctation of the aorta and to specify adjacent anomalies of the aortic arch. But it is not always possible, especially in adults, to obtain images of satisfactory quality. It also allows the demonstration of associated lesions, mainly aortic bicuspidity found in 50 to 85% of patients with coarctation of the aorta [105].

c) Cardiac catheterization:

Until the 1990s [48], cardiac catheterization was considered the reference examination for the anatomic and hemodynamic evaluation of congenital heart disease. However, because of its invasive nature and the improvement in the quality and availability of new imaging techniques, it has lost much of its interest and currently has almost no place. Its use is justified in case of inconclusive or contradictory data and when there is an indication for an associated endovascular procedure as well as for the selective evaluation of the coronary network [79].

d) CT scan:

The major advantages of cardiac CT are its very precise spatial resolution with a shorter acquisition time, the absence of contraindications for patients with implanted pacemakers or defibrillators, and the possibility of visualizing stented vascular structures with less risk of artifacts than with MRI. In the absence of contraindications to MRI, the use of iodinated contrast agents places this examination as a second alternative [79, 106].

Aortic angioscan remains the examination of choice in the morphological diagnosis of coarctation of the aorta, particularly to characterize the location, degree and length of the stenosis, the presence of collateral circulation, the relationship with the left subclavian artery and the association with other cardiovascular anomalies [107]. This information is essential for the choice between reconstructive surgery and transluminal angioplasty [108].

e) Nuclear scintigraphy:

This imaging modality was initially used mainly to assess pulmonary perfusion, left myocardial function, and to quantify the extent of shunting in patients with congenital heart disease. However, it does not provide sufficiently accurate results regarding LV function and dimensions as well as segmental kinetic disturbances. Currently, nuclear scintigraphy has been replaced by MRI.

5. Operative indications:

According to the 2020 European recommendations [109]; Decision-making in GUCH involves accurate diagnosis, timing of intervention, risk assessment and selection of the most appropriate type of intervention. In addition, specific aspects of medical treatment, conditions such as heart failure, pulmonary hypertension and anticoagulant therapy are addressed :

A. Non-cyanogenic congenital heart disease:

a. **AIC-OS:** According to the recommendations of the European Society of Cardiology [109], AIC closure is recommended regardless of symptoms in all patients with signs of right ventricular volume overload and without PAH (no non-invasive signs of PAH or invasive confirmation of pulmonary resistances <3 WU in case of such signs) or LV defect.

Percutaneous closure of aged OS CIAs has become the first therapeutic choice when possible, based on morphology (including stretched diameter <38 mm and sufficient 5-mm rims except on the aortic side). This is the case in 80% of patients. For the remaining 20%, closure will be surgical. However, an important fact in elderly subjects is that the surgical risk must be carefully weighed against the potential benefit of AIC closure.

On the other hand, in patients with impaired left ventricular function (systolic and diastolic), CIA -OS closure may worsen heart failure. These patients should be carefully evaluated and may require pre-interventional testing (balloon occlusion with reassessment of hemodynamics) to decide between complete, fenestrated, or no closure, as an increase in filling pressure due to AIC closure may worsen symptoms and outcome [110].

b. **Partial CAV:** as for CIA-OS, the operative indication is given in case of symptoms or the presence of signs of right ventricular volume overload. The cure is only surgical and it is recommended that it be performed by a surgeon competent in congenital heart disease. For mitral leakage, a plasty is preferable and is indicated for moderate to severe MI in symptomatic patients. However, in asymptomatic patients, surgery is indicated if the MI is severe with LV involvement (LVSD $\geq$ 45 mm and/or LVEF < 60%). If there is no left ventricular function impairment and the operative risk is low, mitral plasty should be considered in the presence of ACFA or PAH > 50 mm Hg.

Indications for reoperation for residual abnormalities are comparable to indications for primary surgery and often relate to left-sided AV valve regurgitation rather than narrowing. It should be noted that these valves are different from normal mitral valves and more difficult to repair [111].

c. **PCA:** the indications for surgery or percutaneous closure are identical to those for CIA-OS. An important fact is that the frequency of ductal calcification can pose a problem for surgery (fragility, need for bypass surgery...) and therefore percutaneous closure is the method of choice, even if cardiac operations are indicated because of other concomitant cardiac lesions [112]. Surgery is then reserved for rare cases with too large a duct or with unfavorable anatomy such as aneurysm formation.

d. **Subvalvular rao:** surgery is indicated in symptomatic patients with a mean LV-AO gradient ≥ 40 mm Hg. Surgery should be considered in asymptomatic patients in case of impaired LV function (LVEF < 50%, significant hypertrophy) or hypotension on exercise.

e. **Aortic Coarctation**: In native CoA, as well as re-coarctation with appropriate anatomy, stenting has become the first line treatment in many centers [113]. The use of covered stents is preferred because of lower short- and long-term complication rates [114].

B. Cyanogenic congenital heart disease:

a. **T4F:** It is recommended that surgical or interventional management of long-term complications of T4F repair be performed only at specialized congenital heart disease centers. Valvulation and/or pulmonary pathway obstruction removal can be performed with a low risk of mortality in patients without heart failure and/or advanced right ventricular dysfunction [115]. The most frequent indication is large PI and optimal timing remains a challenge. In symptomatic patients, pulmonary valvulation is indicated in case of severe PI or stenosis in the middle or tight pulmonary pathway. Normalization of LV size after reintervention becomes unlikely once the indexed telesystolic volume exceeds 80 mL/m2 and telesystolic volume exceeds 160 mL/m2, but this threshold for reintervention may not correlate with clinical benefit. A recent meta-analysis demonstrated that valve replacement can improve symptoms and reduce LV volume, but a survival benefit has yet to be demonstrated [116]. A biological pulmonary valve (xenograft or homograft) appears to have an average lifespan of 10 to 20 years, and future replacement could be performed endovascularly "valve-in-valve".

Percutaneous pulmonary dilatation with often stent implantation is indicated for patients with non-dysplastic valvular PR associated with pulmonary tree stenosis. In contrast, surgery is recommended:

- ✓ On the one hand for patients with subinfundibular or infundibular stenosis with hypoplastic pulmonary annulus and dysplastic valve.
- ✓ On the other hand, for patients with lesions requiring a surgical approach, such as massive PI or severe IT.

The indication for surgical closure of a residual IVC in case of LV volume overload should also be considered.

b. APSO: Untreated patients who survive into adulthood or who have had previous palliative procedures may in fact benefit from modern surgical or interventional procedures. Cases with good-sized confluent PAs and those with large MAPCAs anatomically suitable for unifocalization and who have not developed severe pulmonary vascular disease (due to protective stenosis) should be proposed for surgery. However, many untreated patients may not be suitable for surgery, primarily because of the complexity of their pulmonary vasculature. It is important to understand that although cardiac surgery may improve clinical status or prognosis, it is also a major cause of mortality [117]. Survival depends on the complexity of the pulmonary malformations and the outcome of surgical repair. The survival of palliated patients is significantly lower and has been reported as 60% at 20 years of follow-up. Heart-lung transplantation could be an option for highly selected patients.

c. **Single ventricular hearts**: If the clinical situation is stable, the risk of each type of surgical intervention must be weighed very carefully against the potential benefit. A Fontan operation can be considered only in well-selected patients (low pulmanary resistances; mean PAP <15 mm Hg; good UAV function, no atrioventricular valve regurgitation, and no arrhythmia). "Fenestration" has been performed in some or all cases by some centers to allow shunting of deoxygenated blood to the systemic circulation at the atrial level, aimed at improving cardiac output at the expense of cyanosis. Fontan surgery, when considered late in adults, is not always the best choice because of limited long-term results [118]. For patients with severe cyanosis, with decreased pulmonary blood flow without increased pulmonary resistance, a bidirectional Glenn may be an option. If a systemic-pulmonary shunt is the only option (bidirectional Glenn shunt not sufficient or PAP not low enough for this shunt), the benefit of increased pulmonary blood flow must be weighed against the increased volume load on the ventricular system. For transplantation, iterative sternotomies, aortopulmonary collaterals, and the multisystemic nature are technical and medical challenges and limit outcomes. For UVs with an unprotected or inadequately protected pulmonary pathway, PA banding or recerclage is indicated.

d. **Ebstein's disease**: Surgical repair is recommended in cases of severe and symptomatic IT or with objective deterioration of the patient's exercise capacity. Otherwise, surgical repair can be considered even in asymptomatic patients with progressive dilatation of the right heart chambers or decreased LV systolic function.

   It is recommended that surgical repair be performed by a surgeon experienced in Ebstein's surgery and closure of the IAC is recommended at the time of valve repair if it is expected to be hemodynamically well tolerated.

6. Particularities of iterative surgery :

Iterative surgery exposes patients to the risks of re-entry bleeding, medial infection and postoperative bleeding. These increase the consumption of blood products, the length of hospital stay and could increase early mortality.

i. Iterative surgery and hemorrhagic reentry accident:

The iterative nature of sternotomy and the presence of a VD-AP conduit have been described as the main causes of reentry hemorrhagic events [81]. The origin of the bleeding was a wound of the VD, VD-AP conduit, or aneurysmal pulmonary artery. This rate usually varies between 5% and 10% but in some series it does not exceed 1% [119]. The use of MRI or a profile X-ray allows the posterior relationship of the sternum to be assessed and subsequently minimizes the risk of this accident occurring.

ii. Iterative surgery and surgical site infection:

Several factors favor the occurrence of a surgical site infection. In a study of 1000 cases, Holst and colleagues [120] identified by univariate analysis that the iterative nature of the surgery was a risk factor for infection, but the number of sternotomies in itself had no influence on this risk. In another study [81], none of the 164 patients operated on developed a surgical site infection. These patients were 61% redux and 27% tridux, with a mean number of sternotomies of 2.46.

iii. Iterative surgery and early mortality:

Contrary to what one might think, neither iterative sternotomy nor the occurrence of a re-entrant lesion is a risk factor for early postoperative mortality [119-121]. In a series of 1000 patients [120] with congenital heart disease who received multiple sternotomies, the overall early mortality rate was 3.6%, and multivariate analysis did not identify the number of sternotomies as a risk factor for mortality.

In most of the published series, the iterative nature of this surgery is not an argument delaying or contraindicating the surgical procedure and this in view of the absence of a relationship between early morbidity and mortality and the number of sternotomies the patient has undergone. The respect of certain precautionary measures is sufficient to overcome this inconvenience.

V. Major postoperative complications and early mortality:

1. Early mortality:

Early mortality was significant in recent decades. Dore et al reported an overall early mortality of 7% in a report from 1991 to 1994 [122]. Currently, overall hospital mortality ranges from 1.3% to 6.8% [54,55].

Whenever possible, it should be considered that patients with CC should be referred to highly specialized surgical centers, which carry a lower surgical risk [123,124]. Several scores have been created to estimate the risk in children with CC [124,125]. In contrast, to date, there is no specific risk score for adult patients with CC. In order to establish a global score for surgical risk assessment in this growing population of adult patients, it is mandatory to take into account associated comorbidities, risk factors, the complex pathophysiology in which a procedure is performed as well as the diagnosis leading to surgery.

Although redux surgery carries higher morbidity, Giamberti et al agree that redux surgery can be performed with low risk if approached meticulously in large centers where reoperations are frequently performed [81]. Functional class (NYHA) and QRS duration were also not predictive of higher mortality [126].

2. Major postoperative complications:

Adult congenital heart disease surgery has particular characteristics that differentiate it from congenital cardiac surgery in children and cardiac surgery for acquired diseases in adults: the diversity of anatomoclinic situations and the difficulty of specific surgical techniques are the most important. The presence of multivisceral involvement is frequent in these patients, which complicates anesthesia and the postoperative period [127, 128].

The median length of stay in an intensive care unit varied from one center to another, for example it was 3.9 days in the series by Mello et al [129] and 5 days in the study by Mascio et al [56]. However, it was shorter in the cohort of Putman et al [130] (1.9 days) and Padalino et al [131] (2.3 days).

In a study of 66 patients, Berdat et al [16] identified cyanosis, impaired ventricular function, and prolonged CEC and aortic clamp time as risk factors for postoperative morbidity. Thus, early intervention before the onset of ventricular dysfunction is recommended to reduce the risk of early morbidity and improve outcomes. Indeed, during the study period, there has been a new evolution in the indications and timing of surgery, for example, for pulmonary valve replacement, and a clear trend toward a more prognostic approach, advancing cardiac surgery before overt symptoms develop.

Abarbanell et al. [132] in their review of 234 patients concluded that prolonged CEC and aortic clamping times were significant predictors of morbidity as well as other factors such as preoperative pulmonary or hepatic pathologies and high lactate levels.

Giamberti et al [81] studied 164 reoperated patients with CC and concluded that the duration of the CEC was the most important predictor of morbidity, as it implies the complexity of the procedure.

Preoperative cyanosis is an important risk factor for early and mid-term outcomes in adult CC patients [16, 130, 132]. Long-standing cyanosis is associated with complex cardiac disorders, MAPCAs, hemostasis abnormalities, and cardiac dysfunction [122].

The occurrence of arrhythmias is a well-known complication during the course of congenital heart disease in adulthood often leading to hospitalization. Indeed, the risk of arrhythmias is accentuated due to dilatation of the right atrium, myocardial hypertrophy, and previous surgical interventions [80]. Atrial fibrillation was the most frequent rhythmic complication in our study and the study by Giamberti et al [81].

Anti-arrhythmic pharmacological treatments may offer long-term protection against recurrence in some patients with atrial fibrillation. Surgical ablation may be proposed. However, data on the long-term effect of antiarrhythmic surgery were not available [133].

The difference in reoperation rates between studies may reflect institutional differences in the management of postoperative bleeding [134]. There is little work reporting the incidence of postoperative infections in adults with CC. In a multicenter study by Vida et al, an incidence of 2% was reported [52].

Neurological lesions are known complications in postoperative CC [135]. They may be related to individual patient factors (genetic predisposition, sex), or factors related to operative variables or to the often cyanogenic causative pathology (thrombopathy).

VI. Medium-term evolution:

1. Evolution of functional status:

The subjectivity of dyspnea measurement, the lack of correlation between clinical and ultrasound data and the complicated pathophysiology of this symptom make the interpretation of this evolution and the identification of the variables controlling it rather difficult. In order to remedy this problem, the exercise test coupled with the measurement of gas exchange, although not performed in our study, is the solution of choice. It offers a good correlation between the patient's hemodynamic parameters with maximal oxygen consumption and the anaerobic threshold. It is also an objective and operator independent examination. In a series of 118 patients, Giardini et al [136] showed that maximal oxygen consumption and anaerobic threshold are independent factors of death and hospitalization.

In a study by Geva et al [76] , LV dysfunction and completion of the initial cure at a late age were identified as risk factors for severe dyspnea.

According to Scherptong R W et al [78], patients with QRS duration ≥180ms have less chance to improve their functional classes postoperatively. Vliegen HW et al [74] also found that having NYHA stage IV dyspnea preoperatively decreases the chances of recovery postoperatively. According to Therrien J. [137] and Ferraz C. [138] and their collaborators, the more dilated the VD is, the less reversible the dyspnea will be.

Improvement in functional status was reported in several studies that confirmed the benefits of surgery in the adult population [6, 139]. Nevertheless, the improvement was not significant in either the medium or long term.

2. Evolution of electrical disorders:

a. QRS duration:

QRS duration usually varies between 140 and 180 ms [90, 94, 96, 140].

Decreased QRS duration has been reported in the most recent series [78,138] and subsequently confirms the beneficial role of surgery on ventricular remodeling.

In contrast, widening of the QRS duration after complete cure reflects an abnormally long ventricular depolarization pathway and correlates directly with the degree of right ventricular dilatation. In addition, a QRS duration greater than 180 ms is predictive of sudden death [141].

Many solutions have been proposed to act on the widening of the QRS duration and subsequently on its complications. Examples are the plication of infundibular aneurysms and infundibulectomy [141]. Others have proposed to act in a preventive way by favoring trans-atrial repair and subsequently reducing the size of the widening patch.

A study by Gatzolius et al [77] of 792 patients showed that patients who had a QRS duration ≥ 140ms had their complete cures at a later age than the others.

b. Rhythm disorders:

Arrhythmias occurring immediately postoperatively were associated with a worse clinical outcome. Advanced age, heart failure, significant valvular heart disease, prolonged time on bypass surgery, and myocardial injury during surgery were associated with a high risk of arrhythmia occurrence postoperatively. These findings are consistent with studies of acquired heart disease [142, 143].

This could be explained by the fact that mechanical and electrical remodeling potential is inversely proportional to the age of surgery [77]. Ventricular scar fibrosis and surgery-induced ischemia constitute low conduction areas that favor reentrant VTs [84]. Moreover, the rate of VTs in patients operated for T4F reaches 25% [85].

c. Arrhythmia Solutions:

In order to avoid these arrhythmias and their complications, two approaches exist. The hemodynamic approach consists of repairing the hemodynamic disorders involved, i.e. pulmonary and tricuspid valve dysfunction, and the electrophysiological approach consists of ablation of the reentrant branches, either by endovascular or surgical means [144], as well as the implantation of defibrillators. The biggest problem is to identify patients at risk and therefore candidates for such interventions. This identification can be done via risk stratification. Identified arrhythmia factors are QRS>180ms, advanced age at primary cures, trans-annular patches, LV dilatation, severe PI, complete BAV and non-sporadic ESV [77].

The second means, by far more specific but invasive, is programmed ventricular pacing [145].

According to the study by Karamlou T et al [146], PVR decreases the recurrence of SVRR but not SVRR, hence the importance of concomitant ablation. To minimize the risk of SVRT, some authors advocate preventive cryoablation in cases of significant right atrial dilatation or more than moderate tricuspid insufficiency [137, 144].

3. Evolution of ultrasound parameters:

A clear improvement in echographic parameters was reported by the majority of published studies [94]. In a metanalysis (of 48 studies) published in 2013 [138], Ferraz C et al concluded that there was no significant difference between pre- and postoperative right ventricular function of a pulmonary valve after T4F cure, but this comparison was based on MRI assessment.

Many factors have been correlated with reversibility of right function. Therrien J as well as Ferraz C and colleagues [137,138] demonstrated that right ventricular function is less likely to recover when preoperative FEVD is low: <40% and < 45% respectively. These findings were supported by the work of Ukedem [147].

These results encourage us to focus more on preoperative ventricular function and to try to identify patients with dysfunction at an earlier stage. This implies a more rigorous monitoring and a closer use of MRI and TTE.

Other factors may distort the FEVD measurement, in particular the use of ventriculoplasty techniques [148]. The cure of infundibular aneurysms associated with PVR would cause a postoperative reduction in LV volume that would bias the evolution of FEVD.

- **Evolution of left ventricular function and DV-GV interaction:**

For CCC, there are few studies that report a significant improvement in LVEF, the most recent being that of Tobler [149]. According to him, the change in LVEF depends mainly on its value in pre-operation. Only patients with a pre-PVR LVEF of <45% had significant improvement in LV function. According to Frigiola A. et al [95] increasing FEVD improves left preload and subsequently LVEF. On the other hand, Tzemos N et al [150] showed that the improvement in left ventricular function is related to the decrease in LV-VD asynchrony and subsequently related to the decrease in QRS duration.

VII. Comparison of surgical vs. endovascular treatment:

1. BCP Closure:

A large review of the literature published in 2015 by Lam et al [151], comparing surgery and catheterization shows that there are more reoperations after percutaneous closure, the complication rate is equivalent, and the length of hospital stay is less. However, this study uses data from the last 20 years and techniques have not stopped evolving. Indeed, catheterization is replacing surgery as catheterization techniques and equipment become more sophisticated. This technique is now used in certain centers for very low birth weight premature babies.

2. CIA-OS closures:

Percutaneous closure should be recommended as a first-line procedure because it has the advantage of being less complicated, less invasive than surgery, and less aesthetic damage. Nowadays, the proper diameter of the AIC and the quality of its rims are no longer an important limitation to the use of this technique since the advent of prostheses with an internal diameter of up to 40 mm [152] and the first trials of 3D printing of defects which allowed a more accurate assessment of the diameter of the AIC and its closure even in the presence of insufficient rims on 2D ultrasound [153]. Similarly, the use of fenestrated prostheses has shown good results in patients with significant dilatation of the heart chambers and severe PAH [154]. Conventional surgery also remains a reliable and effective means of correction of AICs with a success rate approaching 100% in many publications.

Mini-thoracotomy represents a less invasive approach that is as safe and effective as sternotomy. It gives results that are as good as those of conventional surgery and does not increase either the operative risk or the postoperative complications [155]. Other techniques are also seeking to become less invasive alternatives to conventional surgery for patients in whom percutaneous closure is impossible, such as totally computer-assisted endoscopic occlusion which offers an excellent aesthetic result [156,157].

3. Coarctation Cure:

Numerous studies have compared the short-, medium-, and long-term efficacy of surgical treatments for coarctation of the aorta and interventional techniques.
A retrospective study conducted in four Quebec centers compared the results of 50 patients treated by interventional means and 30 patients operated on between 1998 and 2004. Immediate results, late and late complications, and long-term outcome were analyzed. There were no deaths in either group after 9 months to 3 years; 32% of reinterventions were reported in the aortic angioplasty with stenting group and none in the surgery group. Hypertension, aneurysms, and transisthmic gradient had a similar incidence in both groups [158].
In 2016 Zhang et al [159] , performed a retrospective study including 92 patients, 39 treated by balloon angioplasty and 53 by surgery. No statistically significant differences in procedural success, transisthmic gradient persistence, complications, and death were observed between angioplasty and surgery.
Comparison of the severity of AH before and after repair by angioplasty or surgery also showed no statistically significant difference.
Cowley CG. et al [160], similarly observed that, compared to surgical patients, patients treated with angioplasty are at significantly higher risk of aneurysm development and consequently the need for reintervention.
It is currently accepted that angioplasty-stenting is the reference treatment for recoarctation in adults and children over 7 years of age, with balloon angioplasty reserved for recoarctation in children over 3 months of age and whose area of coarctation is not too extensive [161].

The study by Walhout R. et al [162] showed a stenting success rate of more than 95% with a complication rate (aortic wounds, dissections and aneurysms) of <10%. Their frequency is lower since the use of covered stents and stents. The medium-term results are comparable to those of conventional surgery. In this study, three patients died after angioplasty, whereas no deaths were observed among patients treated surgically.

4. Pulmonary Valvulation:

There is still no publication concerning the long-term results of percutaneous PVR. But the immediate and medium-term results are very encouraging and far ahead of those of the surgical approach. The intra-hospital mortality rate does not exceed 2%. The rate of major post-procedural complications does not exceed 10% [163, 164]. It should be noted that this comparison is biased by the fact that the choice between the surgical or percutaneous approach is not offered to all patients. Only a portion of the operated patients could have had percutaneous PVR. In order to overcome this, Khanna AD. Et al in 2015 [165] performed a study including 10,000 patients. They selected patients who had undergone surgical PVR and were at the same time eligible for the percutaneous approach (6500 patients from the congenital heart surgery registry and 3500 patients from the adult heart surgery registry). Intra-hospital mortality was 4.1%, and the major complication rate was 20.9%. These results remain quite different from those of the percutaneous approach.

VIII. Quality of life, physical activities and pregnancy:

1. Quality of Life:

As survival of patients with CC has improved in recent years, attention has shifted to more comprehensive measures such as health-related quality of life. There is a large body of data on quality of life in children, adolescents and adults with CC, but their results are divergent [166]. Quality of life is overall good but heterogeneous. This is related to the heterogeneity of CC and the use of different methods to measure QoL [167, 168] and about 10% of patients have a poor QoL.

Factors associated with poor quality of life were: impaired NYHA functional class; not working; advanced age; and being single. Gender, education level and complexity of heart disease were not related to quality of life [169, 170]. However, in a meta-analysis, a significant reduction in quality of life in patients with moderate or complex CC concerned only the physical dimension and not the mental or social dimension [171]. Physical activity, work and sexual life represent fundamental dimensions of quality of life.

2. Physical Activities:

Physical activity is a major issue, directly impacting the quality of life of patients. Nowadays, it is clearly accepted that physical activity is not only beneficial in the long term for quality of life but also in terms of morbidity and mortality [172].

Numerous studies have shown that exercise programs in these patients are both safe and improve physical performance and quality of life [173-175]. Even in patients with PAH, there is a benefit when the physical program is carefully chosen [176, 177]. However, 1/3 of adults with CC are regularly engaged in moderate physical activity and 1/3 have no physical activity at all for a mean age of 26 years [178].

A review specifies the significant differences in physical abilities across the spectrum of CC and the benefit of aerobic activity over a long period of time regardless of CC [179]. These recommendations for physical activity and sport should begin at an early age. It is important that the child and his or her family be informed that a contraindication to sport is exceptionally required, in contrast to the former practice of most cardiopediatricians who prohibited sport.

3. Sexuality, Pregnancy and Contraception:

Sexual activity is an important component of quality of life for the patient and partner. According to AHA recommendations [180], sexual activity is safe for most patients with CC. Women with CC are less sexually active than their peers, however, they are more likely to engage in risky sexual activity such as lack of contraception and use of drugs or alcohol during sex [181].

It is important that this issue be addressed in order to avoid health problems related to risky sexual practices, and unwanted and/or complicated pregnancies in complex heart disease [182]. Indeed, only half of the women contraindicated for pregnancy report having received this information and about half have not been informed about contraceptives, while 28% of patients at high risk of pregnancy do not use contraception during sexual intercourse [183].

The cardiologist and the gynecologist are able to provide expertise on the type of contraception compatible with the patient's CC and on the risks involved in pregnancy.

Most CCs are at low risk, however a NYHA functional class>2, history of arrhythmias, heart failure, stroke, cyanosis, left heart obstruction (aortic or mitral stenosis), are risk factors for maternal and fetal complications during pregnancy [184, 185].

4. Education and professional activity:

According to the literature, patients with CC (<40 years) have worse outcomes compared to a reference group with respect to education, employment and social life. These outcomes are more marked in men [186-188].

Indeed, many studies have shown that the level of education and training achieved by the patient with congenital heart disease is lower than that achieved in the general population. In addition, the employment rate is significantly lower in patients with congenital heart disease compared with that of the reference population, and varies between 59 and 67% [189].

IX. REFERENCES:

1. Dolk, H., Loane, M., Garne, E. & European Surveillance of Congenital Anomalies (EUROCAT) Working Group. Congenital heart defects in Europe: prevalence and perinatal mortality, 2000 to 2005. Circulation 123, 841-849 (2011).

2. Bouma BJ, Sieswerda GT, Post MC, et al. New developments in adult congenital heart disease. Neth Heart J. 2020;28(Suppl 1):44-49. doi:10.1007/s12471-020-01455-5

3. Vida, V., Zanotto, L., Torlai Triglia, L., Zanotto, L., Maruszewski, B., ... Tobota, Z. (2020). Surgery for Adult Patients with Congenital Heart Disease: Results from the European Database. Journal of Clinical Medicine, 9(8), 2493. doi:10.3390/jcm9082493

4. Moller JH, Anderson RC. A 43 - to - 54 year follow-up of 1,000 patients with congenital heart disease. Am J Cardiol 2013;111:1496-500.

5. O'Leary JM, Siddiqi OK, de Ferranti S, et al. The changing demographics of congenital heart disease hospitalizations in the United States, 1998 through 2010. JAMA 2013;309:984-6.

6. Beurtheret S, Tutarel O, Diller GP, et al Contemporary cardiac surgery for adults with congenital heart disease Heart 2017;103:1194-1202.

7. Hoffman JI, Kaplan S, Liberthson RR. Prevalence of congenital heart disease. Am Heart J 2004;147:425-39.

8. Zomer AC, Verheugt CL, Vaartjes I, et al. Surgery in adults with congenital heart disease. Circulation 2011;124:2195-201.

9. Tutarel O, Kempny A, Alonso-Gonzalez R, et al. Congenital heart disease beyond the age of 60: emergence of a new population with high resource utilization, high morbidity, and high mortality. Eur Heart J 2014;35:725-32.

10. Babu-Narayan SV, Diller GP, Gheta RR, et al. Clinical outcomes of surgical pulmonary valve replacement after repair of tetralogy of fallot and potential prognostic value of preoperative cardiopulmonary exercise testing. Circulation 2014;129:18-27.

11. Kim, Y.Y.; Gauvreau, K.; Bacha, E.A.; Landzberg, M.J.; Benavidez, O.J. Risk factors for death after adult congenital heart surgery in pediatric hospitals. Circ. Cardiovasc. Qual. Outcomes 2011, 4, 433-439.

12. Talwar S, Kumar MV, Sreenivas V, Choudhary SK, Sahu M, Airan B. Factors determining outcomes in grown up patients operated for congenital heart diseases. Ann Pediatr Card 2016;9:222-8.

13. Stellin, G.; Vida, V.L.; Padalino, M.A.; Rizzoli, G. European Congenital Heart Surgeons Association. Surgical outcome for congenital heart malformations in the adult age: A multicentric European study. Semin. Thorac. Cardiovasc. Surg. Pediatr. Card. Surg. Annu. 2004, 7, 95-101.

14. Wauthy P, Massaut J, Sanoussi A, Demanet H, Morissens M, et al. Ten-year experience with surgical treatment of adults with congenital cardiac disease. Cardiol Young. 2011 Feb;21(1):39-45.

15. Warnes CA. The adult with congenital heart disease. J Am Coll Cardiol 2005;46:1-8.

16. Berdat PA, Immer F, Pfammatter JP, Carrel T. Reoperations in adults with congenital heart disease: analysis of early outcome. Int J Cardiol. 2004 Feb;93(2-3):239-45. doi: 10.1016/j.ijcard.2003.04.005.

17. Butera G, Romagnoli E, Carminati M, Chessa M, Piazza L, Negura D, et al. Treatment of isolated secundum atrial septal defects: impact of age and defect morphology in 1,013 consecutive patients. Am Heart J. 2008;156(4):706-12.

18. MacDonald ST, Carminati M, Chessa M. Managing adults with congenital heart disease in the catheterization laboratory: state of the art. Expert Rev Cardiovasc Ther. 2010 Dec;8(12):1741-52. doi: 10.1586/erc.10.165.

19. Hughes ML, Maskell G, Goh TH, Wilkinson JL. Prospective comparison of costs and short term health outcomes of surgical versus device closure of atrial septal defect in children. Heart. 2002;88(1):67-70.

20. Karsenty C, Maury P, Blot-Souletie N, Ladouceur M, Leobon B, et al. The medical history of adults with complex congenital heart disease affects their social development and professional activity. Arch Cardiovasc Dis. 2015 Nov;108(11):589-97. doi: 10.1016/j.acvd.2015.06.004.

21. Agarwal S, Sud K, Menon V. Nationwide Hospitalization Trends in Adult Congenital Heart Disease Across 2003-2012. J Am Heart Assoc. 2016 Jan 19;5(1):e002330. doi: 10.1161/JAHA.115.002330.

22. Engelfriet P, Boersma E, Oechslin E, Tijssen J, Gatzoulis MA, et al. The spectrum of adult congenital heart disease in Europe: morbidity and mortality in a 5-year follow-up period. The Euro Heart Survey on adult congenital heart disease. Eur Heart J. 2005 Nov;26(21):2325-33. doi: 10.1093/eurheartj/ehi396

23. Khan A, Gurvitz M. Epidemiology of ACHD: What Has Changed and What is Changing? Prog Cardiovasc Dis. 2018 Sep-Oct;61(3-4):275-281. doi: 10.1016/j.pcad.2018.08.004.

24. Giannakoulas G, Vasiliadis K, Frogoudaki A, Ntellos C, Tzifa A, et al; CHALLENGE investigators. Adult congenital heart disease in Greece: Preliminary data from the CHALLENGE registry. Int J Cardiol. 2017 Oct 15;245:109-13. doi: 10.1016/j.ijcard.2017.07.024.

25. van der Bom T, Mulder BJ, Meijboom FJ, van Dijk AP, Pieper PG, et al. Contemporary survival of adults with congenital heart disease. Heart. 2015 Dec;101(24):1989-95. doi: 10.1136/heartjnl-2015-308144.

26. Aleman-Ortiz OF, Rosas ME, Perez DMR. Epidemiological analysis of the congenital heart disease in adults. J Cardiol Curr Res. 2018;11(2):100-104. DOI: 10.15406/jccr.2018.11.00380

27. G P Diller, P Helm, O Tutarel, U M M Bauer, H Baumgartner, P5479
Optimizing care for adults with congenital heart disease: results of a conjoint analysis based on a nationwide sample of patients included in the German National Register, European Heart Journal, Volume 39, Issue suppl_1, August 2018, ehy566.P5479, Https://doi.org/10.1093/eurheartj/ehy566.P5479

28. Van Bulck L, Luyckx K, Goossens E, Apers S, Kovacs AH, et al. Patient-reported outcomes of adults with congenital heart disease from eight European countries: scrutinizing the association with healthcare system performance. Eur J Cardiovasc Nurs. 2019 Aug;18(6):465-473. doi: 10.1177/1474515119834484.

29. Richard Jonas A. Congenital heart surgery in developing countries. SeminThorac Cardiovasc Surg Pediatr Card Surg Annu 2008;11:3-6.

30. Bannerman CH, Mahalu W. Congenital heart disease in Zimbabwean chil-dren. Ann Trop Paediatr 1998;1:5-12.

31. Awori MN, Ogendo SW. Management pathway for congenital heart diseasein Kennyata National Hospital, Nairobi. East Afr Med J 2007;7:312-7.

32. Mocumbi AO, Lameira E, Yaksh A, Paul L, Ferreira MB, Sidi D. Challenges on the management of congenital heart disease in developing countries. Int J Cardiol. 2011;148:285-8.

33. Kurniawaty J, Widyastuti Y. Outcome of adult congenital heart disease patients undergoing cardiac surgery: clinical experience of dr. Sardjito hospital. BMC Proc. 2019 Dec 16;13(Suppl 11):16. doi: 10.1186/s12919-019-0178-5.

34. Cohen S, Iserin L. Congenital heart disease in adulthood. Blood Thrombosis Vessels. 2014;26(1):23-33. doi:10.1684/stv.2013.

35. Iserin L, Ladouceur M. Adult congenital heart disease: diagnostic conduct. MT Cardio. 2007;3(2):93-101. doi:10.1684/mtc.2007.0087.

36. E. Belli, R. Roussin, C. Planché, A. Serraf, Chirurgie des cardiopathies conénitales à l'âge adulte, EMC-Cardiologie Angéiologie 2 (2005) 191-201

37. Heitz F. Congenital heart disease. EMC AKOS Practical Encyclopedia of Medicine 1998;8:680-94.

38. Cloarec S, Magontier N, Vaillant MC, Paillet C, Chantepie A. Prevalence and distribution of congenital heart diseases in Indre-et-Loire. Evaluation of prenatal diagnosis (1991-1994) [Prevalence and distribution of congenital heart diseases in Indre-et-Loire. Evaluation of prenatal diagnosis (1991-1994). Arch Pediatr. 1999 Oct;6(10):1059-65. French. doi: 10.1016/s0929-693x(00)86979-1.

39. Kverneland LS, Kramer P, Ovroutski S. Five decades of the Fontan operation: A systematic review of international reports on outcomes after univentricular palliation. Congenit Heart Dis. 2018 Mar;13(2):181-193. doi: 10.1111/chd.12570.

40. Chauvaud S. Palliative surgery for tetralogy of Fallot and open interventricular septal pulmonary atresias, EcycMédChir, 2003, 42-810

41. Redo SF, Ecker RR. Intrapericardial Aortic-Pulmonary artery shunt. Circulation. 1963 Oct;28:520-4. doi: 10.1161/01.cir.28.4.520.

42. Nakashima K, Itatani K, Oka N, Kitamura T, Horai T, et al. Pulmonary annulus growth after the modified Blalock-Taussig shunt in tetralogy of Fallot. Ann Thorac Surg. 2014 Sep;98(3):934-40. doi: 10.1016/j.athoracsur.2014.04.083.

43. Kron IL, Nolan SP, Flanagan TL, Gutgesell HP, Muller WH Jr. Pulmonary artery banding revisited. Ann Surg. 1989 May;209(5):642-7; discussion 647. doi: 10.1097/00000658-198905000-00018.

44. Corno AF, Ladusans EJ, Pozzi M, Kerr S. FloWatch versus conventional pulmonary artery banding. J Thorac Cardiovasc Surg. 2007 Dec;134(6):1413-9; discussion 1419-20. doi: 10.1016/j.jtcvs.2007.03.065.

45. Murthy KS, Coelho R, Naik SK, Punnoose A, Thomas W, Cherian KM. Novel techniques of bidirectional Glenn shunt without cardiopulmonary bypass. Ann Thorac Surg. 1999 Jun;67(6):1771-4. doi: 10.1016/s0003-4975(99)00278-7.

46. Chauvaud S. Tricuspid atresia. Fontan procedure and cavo-pulmonary shunts. EMC Chirurgie 2004;1:5-17.

47. Karamlou T, McCrindle BW, Williams WG. Surgery insight: late complications following repair of tetralogy of Fallot and related surgical strategies for management. Nat Clin Pract Cardiovasc Med. 2006 Nov;3(11):611-22. doi: 10.1038/ncpcardio0682.

48. Murphy JG, Gersh BJ, Mair DD, Fuster V, McGoon MD, et al. Long-term outcome in patients undergoing surgical repair of tetralogy of Fallot. N Engl J Med. 1993 Aug 26;329(9):593-9. doi: 10.1056/NEJM199308263290901.

49. Frigiola A, Hughes M, Turner M, Taylor A, Marek J, Giardini A, et al. Physiological and phenotypic characteristics of late survivors of tetralogy of Fallot repair who are free from pulmonary valve replacement. Circulation. 2013; 128 (17):1861-8.

50. Voges I, Fischer G, Scheewe J, Schumacher M, Babu-Narayan SV, Jung O, et al. Restrictive enlargement of the pulmonary annulus at surgical repair of tetralogy of Fallot: 10 years experience with a uniform surgical strategy. Eur J Cardiothorac Surg. 2008;34(5):1041-5.

51. Baumgartner H, Bonhoeffer P, De Groot NM, De Haan F, Deanfield JE, Galie N, et al. Guidelines for the management of grown-up congenital heart disease. Eur Heart J. 2010; 31 (23): 2915-57.

52. Vida VL, Berggren H, Brawn WJ, Daenen W, Di Carlo D, Di Donato R, Lindberg HL, Corno AF, Fragata J, Elliott MJ, Hraska V, Kiraly L, Lacour-Gayet F, Maruszewski B, Rubay J, Sairanen H, Sarris G, Urban A, Van DC, Ziemer G, Stellin G. Risk of surgery for congenital heart disease in the adult: a multicenter European study. Ann Thorac Surg. 2007; 83: 161–168.

53. Daebritz SH. Update in adult congenital cardiac surgery. Pediatr Cardiol. 2007; 28:96-104.

54. Hörer, J.; Vogt, M.; Wottke, M.; Cleuziou, J.; Kasnar-Samprec, J.; Lange, R.; Schreiber, C. Evaluation of the Aristotle complexity models in adult patients with congenital heart disease. Eur. J. Cardiothorac. Surg. 2013, 43, 128–135

55. Marelli, A.J.; Gurvitz, M. From numbers to guidelines. Prog. Cardiovasc. Dis. 2011, 53, 239-246.

56. Mascio, C.E.; Pasquali, S.K.; Jacobs, J.P.; Jacobs, M.L.; Austin, I.I.I.E.H. Outcomes in adult congenital heart surgery: Analysis of the Society of Thoracic Surgeons (STS) Database. J. Thorac. Cardiovasc. Surg. 2011, 142, 1090–1097

57. Williams WG, Ashburn DA, Downar EH. Cardiac reoperations in adults with congenital cardiac surgery. In: Franco KL, Verrier ED (eds.). Advanced Therapy in Cardiac Surgery. BC Decker, London, 2003, pp 263-268.

58. Oechslin EN, Harrison DA, Harris L, Downar E, Webb GD, Siu SS, Williams WG. Reoperation in adults with repair of tetralogy of Fallot: indications and outcomes. J Thorac Cardiovasc Surg. 1999;118:245–251

59. Bertrand Dugardin. Access to loan insurance for adult patients with congenital heart disease. Human Medicine and Pathology. 2010. <dumas-00628995>

60. El-Najdawi EK, Driscoll DJ, Puga FJ, Dearani JA, Spotts BE, Mahoney DW et al. Operation for partial atrioventricular septal defect: a forty-year review. J Thorac Cardiovasc Surg 2000; 119: 880 - 9.

61. Welke KF , Morris CD , King E , Komanapalli C , Reller MD , Ungerleider RM. Population-based perspective of long-term outcomes after surgical repair of partial atrioventricular septal defect. Ann Thorac Surg 2007; 84: 624-8.

62. Stulak JM, Burkhart HM, Dearani JA, Cetta F, Barnes RD, Connolly HM et al. Reoperations after repair of partial atrioventricular septal defect: a 45-year single-center experience. Ann Thorac Surg 2010; 89: 1352 - 9

63. Buratto E , McCrossan B , Galati JC , Bullock A , Kelly A , d'Udekem Y et al . Repair of partial atrioventricular septal defect: a 37-year experience . Eur J Cardiothorac Surg 2015; 47: 796 - 802 .

64. Alexi-Meskishvili V , Hetzer R , Dahnert I , Weng Y , Langr PE . Results of left atrioventricular valve reconstruction after previous correction of atrioventricular septal defects . Eur J Cardiothorac Surg 1997; 12: 460 - 5 .

65. Moran AM , Daebritz S , Keane JF , Mayer JF . Surgical management of mitral regurgitation after repair of endocardial cushion defects: early and midterm results . Circulation 2000; 102 (Suppl III): 160 - 5 .

66. Birim O , van Gameren M , de Jong PL , Witsenburg M , van Osch-Gevers L , Bogers AJJC . Outcome after reoperation for atrioventricular septal defect repair . Interact CardioVasc Thorac Surg 2009; 9: 83 - 8 .

67. Hoohenkerk GJ , Bruggemans EF , Koolbergen DR , Rijlaarsdam ME , Hazekamp MG . Long-term results of reoperation for left atrioventricular valve regurgitation after correction of atrioventricular septal defects . Ann Thorac Surg 2012; 93: 849 - 55 .

68. Malhotra SP1 , Lacour-Gayet F , Mitchell MB , Clarke DR , Dines ML , Campbell DN . Reoperation for left atrioventricular valve regurgitation after atrioventricular septal defect repair . Ann Thorac Surg 2008; 86: 147 - 51 .

69. Hallbergson A, Gauvreau K, Powell AJ, Geva T. Right ventricular remodeling after pulmonary valve replacement: early gains, late losses. Ann Thorac Surg 2015;99(2):660-6.

70. Selly JB, Iriart X, Roubertie F, Mauriat P, Marek J, Guilhon E, et al. Multivariable assessment of the right ventricle by echocardiography in patients with repaired tetralogy of Fallot undergoing pulmonary valve replacement: a comparative study with magnetic resonance imaging. Arch Cardiovasc Dis. 2015;108(1):5-15.

71. Luijten LW, Van Den Bosch E, Duppen N, Tanke R, Roos-Hesselink J, Nijveld A, et al. Long-term outcomes of transatrial-transpulmonary repair of tetralogy of Fallot. Eur J Cardiothorac Surg. 2015;47(3):527-34.

72. Kogon B, Plattner C, Kirshbom P, Kanter K, Leong T, Lyle T, et al. Risk factors for early pulmonary valve replacement after valve disruption in congenital pulmonary stenosis and tetralogy of Fallot. J Thorac Cardiovasc Surg. 2009;138(1):103-8.

73. Muenke M, Kruszka PS, Sable CA, Belmont JW, editors. Congenital Heart Disease: Molecular Genetics, Principles of Diagnosis and Treatment. S. Karger AG; 2015. doi:https://doi.org/10.1159/isbn.978-3-318-03004-4.

74. Vliegen HW, van Straten A, De Roos A, Roest AA, Schoof PH, Zwinderman AH, et al. Magnetic resonance imaging to assess the hemodynamic effects of pulmonary valve replacement in adults late after repair of tetralogy of Fallot. Circulation. 2002;106(13):1703-7.

75. Dimopoulos K, Okonko DO, Diller GP, Broberg CS, Salukhe TV, Babu-Narayan SV, et al. Abnormal ventilatory response to exercise in adults with congenital heart disease relates to cyanosis and predicts survival. Circulation. 2006;113(24):2796-802.

76. Geva T, Sandweiss BM, Gauvreau K, Lock JE, Powell AJ. Factors associated with impaired clinical status in long-term survivors of tetralogy of Fallot repair evaluated by magnetic resonance imaging. J Am Coll Cardiol. 2004;43(6):1068-74.

77. Gatzoulis MA, Balaji S, Webber SA, Siu SC, Hokanson JS, Poile C, et al. Risk factors for arrhythmia and sudden cardiac death late after repair of tetralogy of Fallot: a multicentre study. Lancet. 2000;356(9234):975-81.

78. Scherptong RW, Hazekamp MG, Mulder BJ, Wijers O, Swenne CA, Van Ver Wall EE, et al. Follow-up after pulmonary valve replacement in adults with tetralogy of Fallot: association between QRS duration and outcome. J Am Coll Cardiol. 2010;56(18):1486-92.

79. Valente AM, Cook S, Festa P, Ko HH, Krishnamurthy R, Taylor AM, et al. Multimodality imaging guidelines for patients with repaired tetralogy of Fallot: a report from the american society of echocardiography. J Am Soc Echocardiogr. 2014;27(2):111-41.

80. Le L. Heart failure in adult congenital heart disease. Arch Mal Coeur Vaiss Prat (2018)

81. Giamberti A, Chessa M, Abella R, et al. Morbidity and mortality risk factors in adults with congenital heart disease undergoing cardiac reoperations. Ann Thorac Surg. 2009;88:1284–1289.

82. Kotowycz MA, Therrien J, Ionescu IR, Owens CG, Pilote L, Martucci G, et al. Long-term outcomes after surgical versus transcatheter closure of atrial septal defects in adults. Cardiovasc Interv. 2013;6(5):497-503.

83. Gatzoulis MA, Redington AN, Somerville J, Shore DF. Should atrial septal defects in adults be closed? Ann Thorac Surg. 1996;61(2):657-9.

84. Van Huysduynen BH, Van Straten A, Swenne CA, Maan AC, Van Eck HJ, Schalij MJ, et al. Reduction of QRS duration after pulmonary valve replacement in adult Fallot patients is related to reduction of right ventricular volume. Eur Heart J. 2005;26(9):928-32.

85. Steeds RP, Oakley D. Predicting late sudden death from ventricular arrhythmia in adults following surgical repair of tetralogy of Fallot. QJM. 2003;97(1):7-13.

86. Doughan AR, McConnell ME, Lyle TA, Book WM. Effects of pulmonary valve replacement on QRS duration and right ventricular cavity size late after repair of right ventricular outflow tract obstruction. Am J Cardiol. 2005;95(12):1511-4.

87. Bonnemains L, Stos B, Vaugrenard T, Marie PY, Odille F, Boudjemline Y. Echocardiographic right ventricle longitudinal contraction indices cannot predict ejection fraction in post-operative Fallot children. Eur Heart J Cardiovasc Imaging. 2012;13(3):235-42.

88. Urheim S, Cauduro S, Frantz R, McGoon M, Belohlavek M, Green T, et al. Relation of tissue displacement and strain to invasively determined right ventricular stroke volume. Am J Cardiol. 2005;96(8):1173-8.

89. Kilner PJ. The role of cardiovascular magnetic resonance in adults with congenital heart disease. Prog Cardiovasc Dis. 2011;54(3):295-304.

90. Geva T. Repaired tetralogy of Fallot: the roles of cardiovascular magnetic resonance in evaluating pathophysiology and for pulmonary valve replacement decision support. J Cardiovasc Magn Reson. 2011;13(17):9.

91. Promphan W, Wonglikhitpanya T, Katanyuwong P, Siripornpitak S. A comparative study: right ventricular assessment in post-repaired tetralogy of Fallot patients by echocardiogram with cardiac magnetic resonance imaging. J Med Assoc Thai. 2014;97 Suppl 6:S232-S8.

92. Schwerzmann M, Samman AM, Salehian O, Holm J, Provost Y, Webb GD, et al. Comparison of echocardiographic and cardiac magnetic resonance imaging for assessing right

ventricular function in adults with repaired tetralogy of Fallot. Am J Cardiol. 2007; 99 (11): 1593-7.

93. Villafane J, Feinstein JA, Jenkins KJ, Vincent RN, Walsh EP, Dubin AM, et al. Hot topics in tetralogy of Fallot. J Am Coll Cardiol. 2013;62(23):2155-66.

94. Oosterhof T, Van Straten A, Vliegen HW, Meijboom FJ, Van Dijk AP, Spijkerboer AM, et al. Preoperative thresholds for pulmonary valve replacement in patients with corrected tetralogy of Fallot using cardiovascular magnetic resonance. Circulation. 2007;116(5):545-51.

95. Frigiola A, Tsang V, Bull C, Coats L, Khambadkone S, Derrick G, et al. Biventricular response after pulmonary valve replacement for right ventricular outflow tract dysfunction: is age a predictor of outcome? Circulation. 2008;118 Suppl 14:S182-S90.

96. Buechel ER, Dave HH, Kellenberger CJ, Dodge-Khatami A, Pretre R, Berger F, et al. Remodelling of the right ventricle after early pulmonary valve replacement in children with repaired tetralogy of Fallot: assessment by cardiovascular magnetic resonance. Eur Heart J. 2005;26(24):2721-7.

97. Geva T. Indications for pulmonary valve replacement in repaired tetralogy of Fallot: the quest continues. Circulation. 2013;128(17):1855-7.

98. Therrien J, Provost Y, Merchant N, Williams W, Colman J, Webb G. Optimal timing for pulmonary valve replacement in adults after tetralogy of Fallot repair. Am J Cardiol. 2005;95(6):779-82.

99. Lee C, Kim YM, Lee CH, Kwak JG, Park CS, Song JY, et al. Outcomes of pulmonary valve replacement in 170 patients with chronic pulmonary regurgitation after relief of right ventricular outflow tract obstruction: implications for optimal timing of pulmonary valve replacement. J Am Coll Cardiol. 2012;60(11):1005-14.

100. Koestenberger M, Nagel B, Ravekes W, Everett AD, Stueger HP, Heinzl B, et al. Tricuspid annular plane systolic excursion and right ventricular ejection fraction in pediatric and adolescent patients with tetralogy of Fallot, patients with atrial septal defect and age-matched normal subjects. Clin Res Cardiol. 2011;100(1):67-75.

101. Kurkluoglu M, John AS, Cross R, Chung D, Yerebakan C, Zurakowski D, et al. Should tricuspid annuloplasty be performed with pulmonary valve replacement for pulmonary regurgitation in repaired tetralogy of Fallot? Semin Thorac Cardiovasc Surg. 2015;27(2):159-65.

102. Havasi K, Ambrus N, Kalapos A, Forster T, Nemes A. The role of echocardiography in the management of adult patients with congenital heart disease following operative treatment. Cardiovasc Diagn Ther. 2018;8(6):771-779. doi:10.21037/cdt.2018.09.11

103. Rao PS, Harris AD. Recent advances in managing septal defects: atrial septal defects. F1000Res 2017; 6:2042. 10. 12688/f1000research.11844.1

104. Martin SS, Shapiro EP, Mukherjee M. Atrial Septal Defects - Clinical Manifestations, Echo Assessment, and Intervention. Clin Med Insights Cardiol 2015;8:93-8

105. Chen Z, Zhou Y, Wang J, Liu X, Ge S, He Y. Modeling of coarctation of aort1a in human fetuses using 3D/4D fetal echocardiography and computational fluid dynamics. Echocardiography. dec 2017;34(12):1858 66.

106. Huang F, Chen Q, Huang W, Wu H, Li W, Lai Q. Diagnosis of Congenital Coarctation of the Aorta and Accompanying Malformations in Infants by Multi-Detector Computed Tomography Angiography and Transthoracic Echocardiography: A Chinese Clinical Study. Med Sci Monit. 16 May 2017;23:2308 14.

107. Zhao Q, Shi K, Yang Z, Diao K, Xu H, Liu X, et al. Predictors of aortic dilation in patients with coarctation of the aorta: evaluation with dual-source computed tomography. BMC Cardiovasc Disord. dec 2018;18(1):124.

108. Nance JW, Ringel RE, Fishman EK. Coarctation of the aorta in adolescents and adults: A review of clinical features and CT imaging. J Cardiovasc Comput Tomogr. Jan 2016;10(1):1 12.

109. Baumgartner H, De Backer J, Babu-Narayan SV, Budts W, Chessa M, et al; ESC Scientific Document Group. 2020 ESC Guidelines for the management of adult congenital heart disease. Eur Heart J. 2021 Feb 11;42(6):563-645. doi: 10.1093/eurheartj/ehaa554.

110. Tadros VX, Asgar AW. Atrial septal defect closure with left ventricular dysfunction. EuroIntervention. 2016 May 17;12 Suppl X:X13-X17. doi: 10.4244/EIJV12SXA3.

111. Malhotra SP, Lacour-Gayet F, Mitchell MB, Clarke DR, Dines ML, Campbell DN. Reoperation for left atrioventricular valve regurgitation after atrioventricular septal defect repair. Ann Thorac Surg 2008;86:147151; discussion 151142

112. Fisher RG, Moodie DS, Sterba R, Gill CC. Patent ductus arteriosus in adults-long-term follow-up: nonsurgical versus surgical treatment. J Am Coll Cardiol 1986;8:280284

113. Ringel RE, Vincent J, Jenkins KJ, Gauvreau K, Moses H, Lofgren K, Usmani K. Acute outcome of stent therapy for coarctation of the aorta: results of the coarctation of the aorta stent trial. Catheter Cardiovasc Interv 2013;82:503510

114. Taggart NW, Minahan M, Cabalka AK, Cetta F, Usmani K, Ringel RE, COAST II Investigators. Immediate outcomes of covered stent placement for treatment or prevention of aortic wall injury associated with coarctation of the aorta (COAST II). JACC Cardiovasc Interv 2016;9:484493

115. Babu-Narayan SV, Diller GP, Gheta RR, Bastin AJ, Karonis T, et al. Clinical outcomes of surgical pulmonary valve replacement after repair of tetralogy of Fallot and potential prognostic value of preoperative cardiopulmonary exercise testing. Circulation 2014;129:1827

116. Mongeon FP, Ben Ali W, Khairy P, Bouhout I, Therrien J et al. Pulmonary valve replacement for pulmonary regurgitation in adults with tetralogy of Fallot: a meta-analysisa report for the writing committee of the 2019 update of the Canadian Cardiovascular Society Guidelines for the management of adults with congenital heart disease. Can J Cardiol 2019;35:17721783

117. Belli E, Mace L, Ly M, Dervanian P, Pineau E, Roussin R, Lebret E, Serraf A. surgical management of pulmonary atresia with ventricular septal defect in late adolescence and adulthood. Eur J Cardiothorac Surg 2007;31:236241

118. Kim SJ, Kim WH, Lim HG, Lee JY. Outcome of 200 patients after an extracardiac Fontan procedure. J Thorac Cardiovasc Surg 2008;136:108116

119. Morales DL, Zafar F, Arrington KA, Gonzalez SM, McKenzie ED, Heinle JS, et al. Repeat sternotomy in congenital heart surgery: no longer a risk factor. Ann Thorac Surg. 2008;86(3):897-902

120. Holst KA, Dearani JA, Burkhart HM, Connolly HM, Warnes CA, Li Z, et al. Risk factors and early outcomes of multiple reoperations in adults with congenital heart disease. Ann Thorac Surg. 2011;92(1):122-8.

121. Kirshbom PM, Myung RJ, Simsic JM, Kramer ZB, Leong T, Kogon BE, et al. One thousand repeat sternotomies for congenital cardiac surgery: risk factors for reentry injury. Ann Thorac Surg. 2009;88(1):158-61.

122. Dore A, Glancy DL, Stone S, Menashe VD, Somerville J. Cardiac surgery for grownup -congenital heart patients: Survey of 307 consecutive operations from 1991 to 1994. Am J Cardiol 1997;80:90613-.

123. Karamlou, T.; Diggs, S.D.; Ungerleider, R.M.; Welke, K.F. Adults or Big Kids: What Is the Ideal Clinical Environment for Management of Grown-Up Patients with Congenital Heart Disease? Ann. Thorac. Surg. 2010, 90, 573–579

124. Fuchs, M.; Schibilsky, D.; Zeh, W.; Berchtold-Herz, M.; Beyersdorf, F.; Siepe, M. Does the heart transplant have a future? Eur. J. Cardiothorac. Surg. 2019, 55, i38-i48

125. O'Brien, S.M.; Clarke, D.R.; Jacobs, J.P.; Jacobs, M.L.; Lacour-Gayet, F.G.; Pizarro, C; Welke, K.F.; Maruszewski, B.; Tobota, Z.; Miller, W.J.; et al. An empirically based tool

for analyzing mortality associated with congenital heart surgery. J. Thorac. Cardiovasc. Surg. 2009, 138, 1139–1153

126. Discigil B, Dearani JA, Puga FJ, Schaff HV, Hagler DJ, Warnes CA, et al. Late pulmonary valve replacement after repair of tetralogy of Fallot. J Thorac Cardiovasc Surg. 2001;121(2):344-51.

127. Baum VC. The adult with congenital heart disease. J Cardiothorac Vasc Anesth 1996;10:261-82.

128. Drink water DC. The surgical management of congenital heart disease in the adult. Prog Pediatr Cardiol 2003;17: 81-9.

129. Mello GA, Carvalho JL, Baucia JA, MagalhaesFilho J. Adults with congenital heart disease undergoing first surgery: Prevalence and outcomes at a tertiary hospital. Rev Bras Cir Cardiovasc 2012;27:529 34.

130. Putman LM, vanGameren M, Meijboom FJ, de Jong PL, Roos Hesselink JW, Witsenburg M, et al. Seventeen years of adult congenital heart surgery: A single center experience. Eur J Cardiothoracic Surg 2009;36:96 104.

131. Padalino MA, Speggiorin S, Rizzoli G, Crupi G, Vida VL, Bernabei M, et al. Midterm results of surgical intervention for congenital heart disease in adults: An Italian multicentre study. J Thorac Cardiovasc Surg. 2007;134:106 13.

132. Abarbanell GL, Goldberg CS, Devaney EJ, Ohye RG, Bove EL, Charpie JR. Early surgical morbidity and mortality in adults with congenital heart disease: The University of Michigan experience. Congenit Heart Dis 2008;3:829-.

133. Walsh EP, Cecchin F. Arrhythmias in adult patients with congenital heart disease. Circulation. 2007; 115:534–545.

134. Dos L, Dadashev A, Tanous D, et al. Pulmonary valve replacement in repaired tetralogy of Fallot: determinants of early postoperative adverse outcomes. J Thorac Cardiovasc Surg. 2009;138:553–559

135. Ballweg JA, Wernovsky G, Gaynor JW. Neurodevelopmental outcomes following congenital heart surgery. Pediatr Cardiol 2007;28:126-33.

136. Giardini A, Specchia S, Tacy TA, Coutsoumbas G, Gargiulo G, Donti A, et al. Usefulness of cardiopulmonary exercise to predict long-term prognosis in adults with repaired tetralogy of Fallot. Am J Cardiol. 2007;99(10):1462-7.

173. Therrien J, Siu SC, McLaughlin PR, Liu PP, Williams WG, Webb GD. Pulmonary valve replacement in adults late after repair of tetralogy of Fallot: are we operating too late? J Am Coll Cardiol. 2000;36(5):1670-5.

138. Ferraz Cavalcanti PE, Sa MP, Santos CA, Esmeraldo IM, De Escobar RR, De Menezes AM, et al. Pulmonary valve replacement after operative repair of tetralogy of Fallot: meta-analysis and meta-regression of 3,118 patients from 48 studies. J Am Coll Cardiol. 2013;62(23):2227-43.

139. Abouelella RS, Habib EA, AlHalees ZY, Alanazi MN, Ibhais ME, Alwadai AH. Outcome of cardiac surgery in adults with congenital heart disease: A single center experience. J Saudi Heart Assoc. 2019;31(3):145-150. doi:10.1016/j.jsha.2019.05.003

140. Gengsakul A, Harris L, Bradley TJ, Webb GD, Williams WG, Siu SC, et al. The impact of pulmonary valve replacement after tetralogy of Fallot repair: a matched comparison. Eur J Cardiothorac Surg. 2007;32(3):462-8.

141. Therrien J, Siu SC, Harris L, Dore A, Niwa K, Janousek J, et al. Impact of pulmonary valve replacement on arrhythmia propensity late after repair of tetralogy of Fallot. Circulation. 2001;103(20):2489-94.

142. Delaney JW, Moltedo JM, Dziura JD, et al. Early postoperative arrhythmias after pediatric cardiac surgery. J Thorac Cardiovasc Surg 2006;131:1296-300

143. Almassi GH, Schowalter T, Nicolosi AC, et al. Atrial fibrillation after cardiac surgery: a major morbid event? Ann Surg 1997;226:501-11.

144. Kopf GS, Mello DM, Kenney KM, Moltedo J, Rollinson NR, Snyder CS. Intraoperative radiofrequency ablation of the atrium: effectiveness for treatment of supraventricular tachycardia in congenital heart surgery. Ann Thorac Surg. 2002;74(3):797-804.

145. Khairy P, Landzberg MJ, Gatzoulis MA, Lucron H, Lambert J, Marcon F, et al. Value of programmed ventricular stimulation after tetralogy of Fallot repair: a multicenter study. Circulation. 2004;109(16):1994-2000.

146. Karamlou T, McCrindle BW, Williams WG. Surgery insight: late complications following repair of tetralogy of Fallot and related surgical strategies for management. Nat Clin Pract Cardiovasc Med. 2006;3(11):611-22.

147. Udekem Y. Is long-standing pulmonary regurgitation that deleterious? Some lessons from the past. Heart. 2017;103(4):260-1.

148. Frigiola A, Giamberti A, Chessa M, Di Donato M, Abella R, Foresti S, et al. Right ventricular restoration during pulmonary valve implantation in adults with congenital heart disease. Eur J Cardiothorac Surg. 2006;29 Suppl 1:S279-S85.

149. Tobler D, Crean AM, Redington AN, Van Arsdell GS, Caldarone CA, Nanthakumar K, et al. The left heart after pulmonary valve replacement in adults late after tetralogy of Fallot repair. Int J Cardiol. 2012;160(3):165-70.

150. Tzemos N, Harris L, Carasso S, Subira LD, Greutmann M, Provost Y, et al. Adverse left ventricular mechanics in adults with repaired tetralogy of Fallot. Am J Cardiol. 2009;103(3):420-5

151. Brunetti MA, Ringel R, Owada C, Coulson J, Jennings JM, Hoyer MH, et al. Percutaneous closure of patent ductus arteriosus: a multiinstitutional registry comparing multiple devices. Catheter Cardiovasc Interv Off J Soc Card Angiogr Interv. 2010 Nov1;76(5):696-702

152. Lopez K, Dalvi BV, Balzer D, Bass JL, Momenah T, Cao QL, et al. Transcatheter closure of large secundum atrial septal defects using the 40 mm amplatzer septal occluder: results of an international registry. Catheter Cardiovasc Interv. 2005;66(4):580-4.

153. Wang Z, Liu Y, Xu Y, Gao C, Chen Y, Luo H. Three-dimensional printing-guided percutaneous transcatheter closure of secundum atrial septal defect with rim deficiency: first-in-human series. Cardiol J. 2016;23(6):599-603.

154. Donald ST, Arcidiacono C, Butera G. Fenestrated amplatzer atrial septal defect occluder in an elderly patient with restrictive left ventricular physiology. Heart. 2011;97(5):438

155. Giamberti A, Mazzera E, Di chiara L, Ferretti E, Pasquini L, Di donato RM. Right submammary minithoracotomy for repair of congenital heart defects. Eur J Cardiothorac Surg . 2000;18(6):678-82.

156. Argenziano M, Oz MC, Kohmoto T, Morgan J, Dimitui J, Mongero L, et al. Totally endoscopic atrial septal defect repair with robotic assistance. Circulation. 2003;108(24):191-4.

157. Torracca L, Ismeno G, Alfieri O. Totally endoscopic computer-enhanced atrial septal defect closure in six patients. Ann Thorac Surg. 2001;72(4):1354-7.

158. Rodés-Cabau J, Miró J, Dancea A, Ibrahim R, Piette E, Lapierre C, et al. Comparison of surgical and transcatheter treatment for native coarctation of the aorta in patients ≥1 year old. The Quebec Native Coarctation of the Aorta Study. Am Heart J. Jul 2007;154(1):186 92.

159. Zhang H, Ye M, Chen G, Liu F, Wu L, Jia B. A comparison of balloon angioplasty of native coarctation versus surgical repair for short segment coarctation associated with ventricular septal defect-a single-center retrospective review of 92 cases. J Thorac Dis. August 2016;8(8):2046 52.

160. Cowley CG, Orsmond GS, Feola P, McQuillan L, Shaddy RE. Long-Term, Randomized Comparison of Balloon Angioplasty and Surgery for Native Coarctation of the Aorta in Childhood. Circulation. June 28, 2005;111(25):3453 6.

161. Pascual-Tejerina V, Sánchez-Recalde A, Garzón G, Zamorano JL. A novel transcatheter technique to treat of post-coarctation aneurysm with device occlusion of the aortic arch and descending aorta in a patient with an extra-anatomic bypass. Eur Heart J. 27 Sep 2019;ehz670

162. Walhout RJ, Lekkerkerker JC, Oron GH, Bennink GBWE, Meijboom EJ, Comparison of surgical repair with balloon angioplasty for native coarctation in patients from 3 months to 16 years of age, Eur J Cardiothorac Surg. May 2004;25(5):722 7

163. Haas NA, Carere RG, Kretschmar O, Horlick E, Rodes-Cabau J, De Wolf D, et al. Early outcomes of percutaneous pulmonary valve implantation using the Edwards SAPIEN XT transcatheter heart valve system. Int J Cardiol. 2018;250(24):86-91.

164. Fraisse A, Aldebert P, Malekzadeh-Milani S, Thambo JB, Piechaud JF, Aucoururier P, et al. Melody transcatheter pulmonary valve implantation: results from a French registry. Arch Cardiovasc Dis. 2014;107(11):607-14.

165. Khanna AD, Hill KD, Pasquali SK, Wallace AS, Masoudi FA, Jacobs ML, et al. Benchmark outcomes for pulmonary valve replacement using the society of thoracic surgeons databases. Ann Thorac Surg. 2015;100(1):138-45.

166. Fteropoulli T, Stygall J, Cullen S, Deanfield J, Newman SP, Quality of life of adult congenital heart disease patients: a systematic review of the literature, Cardiol Young. 2013 Aug; 23(4):473-85. doi: 10.1017/S1047951112002351. Epub 2013 Feb 6. PMID: 23388149.

167. Apers S, Luyckx K, Moons P, Quality of life in adult congenital heart disease: what do we already know and what do we still need to know, Curr Cardiol Rep. 2013 Oct;15(10):407. doi: 10.1007/s11886-013-0407-x. PMID: 23955787.

168. Bratt EL, Moons P, Forty years of quality-of-life research in congenital heart disease: Temporal trends in conceptual and methodological rigor, Int J Cardiol. 2015 Sep 15; 195:1-6. doi: 10.1016/j.ijcard.2015.05.070. Epub 2015 May 15. PMID: 26011404.

169. Singh JA, Satele D, Pattabasavaiah S, Buckner JC, Sloan JA, Normative data and clinically significant effect sizes for single-item numerical linear analog self-assessment (LASA) scales, Health Qual Life Outcomes. 2014 Dec 18;12:187. doi: 10.1186/s12955-014-0187-z. PMID: 25519478; PMCID: PMC4302440.

170 Philip Moons, Kristien Van Deyk, Kristel Marquet, Els Raes, Leentje De Bleser et al, Individual quality of life in adults with congenital heart disease: a paradigm shift, European

Heart Journal, Volume 26, Issue 3, February 2005, Pages 298-307, https://doi.org/10.1093/eurheartj/ehi054

171. Philip Moons, Kristien Van Deyk, Leentje De Bleser, Kristel Marquet, Els Raes et al, Quality of life and health status in adults with congenital heart disease: a direct comparison with healthy counterparts, European journal of cardiovascular prevention and rehabilitation, Volume 13, Issue 3, 1 June 2006, Pages 407-413, https://doi.org/10.1097/01.hjr.0000221864.19415.a0

172. Peter C. Kahr, Robert M. Radke, Stefan Orwat, Helmut Baumgartner, Gerhard-Paul Diller, Analysis of associations between congenital heart defect complexity and health-related quality of life using a meta-analytic strategy, International Journal of Cardiology, Volume 199, 2015, Pages 197-203, ISSN 0167-5273, https://doi.org/10.1016/j.ijcard.2015.07.045

173. Piepoli MF, Davos C, Francis DP, Coats AJ, ExTraMATCH Collaborative, Exercise training meta-analysis of trials in patients with chronic heart failure (ExTraMATCH), BMJ. 2004 Jan 24; 328(7433):189. doi: 10.1136/bmj.37938.645220.EE. Epub 2004 Jan 16. PMID: 14729656; PMCID: PMC318480.

174. Jaspal S. Dua, Ashley R. Cooper, Kenneth R. Fox, A. Graham Stuart, Exercise training in adults with congenital heart disease: Feasibility and benefits, International Journal of Cardiology, Volume 138, Issue 2, 2010, Pages 196-205, ISSN 0167-5273, https://doi.org/10.1016/j.ijcard.2009.01.038.
(https://www.sciencedirect.com/science/article/pii/S0167527309000485)

175. Fredriksen PM, Kahrs N, Blaasvaer S, Sigurdsen E, Gundersen O et al, Effect of physical training in children and adolescents with congenital heart disease, Cardiology in the Young. Cambridge University Press; 2000;10(2):107-14.

176. Therrien J, Fredriksen P, Walker M, Granton J, Reid GJ et al, A pilot study of exercise training in adult patients with repaired tetralogy of Fallot, Can J Cardiol. 2003 May;19(6):685-9. PMID: 12772019.

177. Newman JH, Robbins IM, Exercise training in pulmonary hypertension: implications for the evaluation of drug trials, Circulation. 2006 Oct 3;114(14):1448-9. doi: 10.1161/CIRCULATIONAHA.106.649079. PMID: 17015802.

178. Desai SA, Channick RN, Exercise in patients with pulmonary arterial hypertension, J Cardiopulm Rehabil Prev. 2008 Jan-Feb;28(1):12-6. doi: 10.1097/01.HCR.0000311502.57022.73. Erratum in: J Cardiopulm Rehabil Prev. 2008 Mar-Apr;28(2):table of contents. PMID: 18277824.

179. Swan L, Hillis WS, Exercise prescription in adults with congenital heart disease: a long way to go, Heart. 2000 Jun;83(6):685-7. doi: 10.1136/heart.83.6.685. PMID: 10814630; PMCID: PMC1760864.

180. Kempny A, Dimopoulos K, Uebing A, Moceri P, Swan L et al, Reference values for exercise limitations among adults with congenital heart disease. Relation to activities of daily life-single center experience and review of published data, Eur Heart J. 2012 Jun; 33(11):1386-96. doi: 10.1093/eurheartj/ehr461. Epub 2011 Dec 23. PMID: 22199119.

181. Levine, G. N., Steinke, E. E., Bakaeen, F. G., Bozkurt, B., Cheitlin, M. D. et al, Sexual Activity and Cardiovascular Disease: A Scientific Statement From the American Heart Association, Circulation, 125(8), 1058-1072. doi:10.1161/cir.0b013e3182447787

182. Graham J. Reid, Samuel C. Siu, Brian W. McCrindle, M. Jane Irvine, Gary D. Webb, Sexual behavior and reproductive concerns among adolescents and young adults with congenital heart disease, International Journal of Cardiology, Volume 125, Issue 3, 2008, Pages 332-338, ISSN 0167-5273, https://doi.org/10.1016/j.ijcard.2007.02.040. (https://www.sciencedirect.com/science/article/pii/S0167527307005311)

183. Miner PD, Canobbio MM, Pearson DD, Schlater M, Balon Y et al, Contraceptive Practices of Women With Complex Congenital Heart Disease, Am J Cardiol. 2017 Mar 15;119(6):911-915. doi: 10.1016/j.amjcard.2016.11.047. Epub 2016 Dec 18. PMID: 28087052.

184. Vigl M, Kaemmerer M, Seifert-Klauss V, Niggemeyer E, Nagdyman N et al, Contraception in women with congenital heart disease, Am J Cardiol. 2010 Nov 1;106(9):1317-21. doi: 10.1016/j.amjcard.2010.06.060. PMID: 21029831.

185. Swan L. Congenital heart disease in pregnancy. Best Pract Res Clin Obstet Gynaecol. 2014 May;28(4):495-506. doi: 10.1016/j.bpobgyn.2014.03.002. Epub 2014 Mar 13. PMID: 24675221.

186. Ladouceur M, Benoit L, Radojevic J, Basquin A, Dauphin C et al, Pregnancy outcomes in patients with pulmonary arterial hypertension associated with congenital heart disease, Heart. 2017 Feb 15;103(4):287-292. doi: 10.1136/heartjnl-2016-310003. Epub 2016 Aug 10. PMID: 27511447.

187. Zomer AC, Vaartjes I, Uiterwaal CS, van der Velde ET, Sieswerda GJ et al, Social burden and lifestyle in adults with congenital heart disease, Am J Cardiol. 2012 Jun 1;109(11):1657-63. doi: 10.1016/j.amjcard.2012.01.397. Epub 2012 Mar 23. PMID: 22444325.

188. Kamphuis M, Vogels T, Ottenkamp J, Van Der Wall EE, Verloove-Vanhorick SP et al, Employment in adults with congenital heart disease, Arch Pediatr Adolesc Med. 2002 Nov;156(11):1143-8. doi: 10.1001/archpedi.156.11.1143. PMID: 12413345.

189. Nieminen H, Sairanen H, Tikanoja T, Leskinen M, Ekblad H et al, Long-term results of pediatric cardiac surgery in Finland: education, employment, marital status, and parenthood, Pediatrics. 2003 Dec;112(6 Pt 1):1345-50. doi: 10.1542/peds.112.6.1345. PMID: 14654608.

TABLE OF CONTENTS

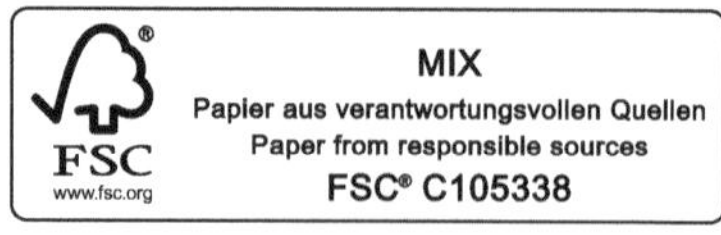

Printed by Books on Demand GmbH, Norderstedt / Germany